Leukaemia Diet Cookbook

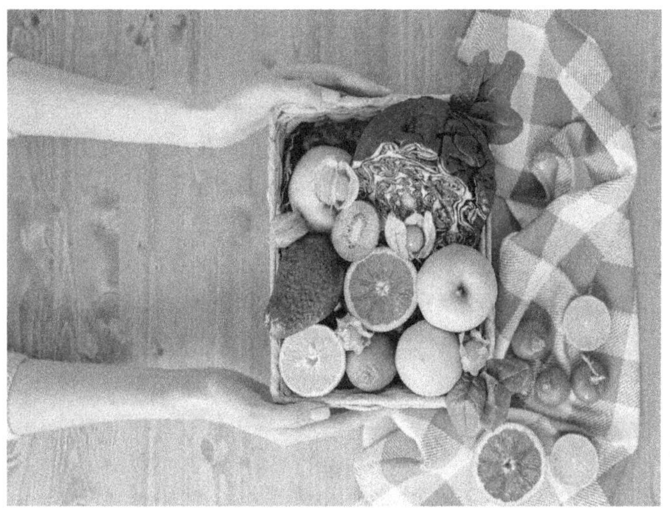

Strategies for Healthy Eating and Delicious Recipes for People down with Cancer

Isaac Hendricks

Table of Contents

INTRODUCTION

Understanding Leukaemia and Dietary Needs

Leukaemia is a type of cancer that affects the blood-forming cells in the bone marrow. It causes an overproduction of abnormal white blood cells, which can lead to a variety of symptoms, including fatigue, fever, and easy bruising or bleeding. While there is no cure for leukaemia, treatment options such as chemotherapy, radiation therapy, and stem cell transplant can help manage the disease and improve overall health.

In addition to medical treatments, dietary changes can also play a role in managing leukaemia. Here are some things to understand about leukaemia and dietary needs:

1. Nutrition is important: People with leukaemia may experience a loss of appetite, nausea, or mouth sores, which can make it difficult to eat enough to maintain a healthy weight. However, getting enough nutrients is crucial for managing the disease and supporting overall health.

2. Consult with a healthcare team: It's important to talk to a healthcare team about dietary needs during leukaemia treatment. Different types of leukaemia and treatments may have different dietary recommendations. For example, people undergoing chemotherapy may need to avoid certain foods that could interact with the medication.

3. Focus on whole foods: Whole foods such as fruits, vegetables, whole grains, and lean proteins can provide the nutrients needed to manage leukaemia. These foods are also generally lower in fat and calories than processed foods, which can be helpful for maintaining a healthy weight during treatment.

4. Stay hydrated: Dehydration is common during leukaemia treatment due to increased urination and vomiting. Drinking plenty of water and other hydrating beverages can help prevent dehydration and support overall health.

5. Manage side effects: Leukaemia treatment can cause side effects such as mouth sores, diarrhoea, or constipation. Dietary changes such as avoiding spicy or acidic foods for mouth sores or increasing fibre intake for constipation can help manage these side effects.

6. Consider supplements: In some cases, people with leukaemia may need to take supplements to ensure they are getting enough nutrients. For example, vitamin B12 is important for people undergoing chemotherapy that affects the stomach or intestines, as these treatments can interfere with absorption of this vitamin from food sources.

In summary, understanding the dietary needs during leukaemia treatment involves working closely with a healthcare team to develop an individualised nutrition plan that addresses specific needs and side effects associated with the disease and treatment options. By focusing on whole foods, staying hydrated, managing side effects, and considering supplements as needed, people with leukaemia can support overall health and well-being during treatment.

The Importance of a Healthy Diet During Treatment

Leukaemia is a blood malignancy that affects the bone marrow. Treatment for leukaemia can be intense and often includes chemotherapy, radiation therapy, and stem cell transplants. While these treatments are necessary for managing the disease, they can also take a toll on the body, causing side effects such as nausea, fatigue, and weight loss. That's why it's crucial to maintain a healthy diet during treatment to support the body's healing process and manage these side effects. In this cookbook, we will explore the importance of a healthy diet during leukaemia treatment and provide recipes that are nutritious, delicious, and easy to prepare.

1. Maintain a Balanced Diet:

A balanced diet is essential for maintaining good health during leukaemia treatment. This means consuming a variety of foods from each food group, including fruits, vegetables, whole grains, lean proteins, and healthy fats. A balanced diet provides the body with the necessary nutrients to support healing and manage side effects such as fatigue and weight loss.

2. Manage Nausea:

Nausea is a common side effect of leukaemia treatment. To manage nausea, it's essential to consume small, frequent meals throughout the day instead of large meals. This helps prevent feelings of fullness and discomfort. It's also important to choose foods that are easy to digest and avoid foods that are spicy or greasy.

3. Manage Fatigue:

Fatigue is another common side effect of leukaemia treatment. To manage fatigue, it's essential to consume foods that are rich in iron and vitamin B12, as these nutrients help support energy levels. Foods such as lean red meat, poultry, fortified cereals, and leafy green vegetables are excellent sources of iron and vitamin B12. It's also critical to stay hydrated during the day by drinking plenty of water.

Weight loss is a common side effect of leukaemia treatment due to decreased appetite and malabsorption of nutrients. To manage weight loss, it's essential to consume high-calorie foods that are nutrient-dense. Foods such as avocados, nuts, seeds, and dried fruits are excellent sources of calories and nutrients. It's also important to consume foods that are easy to digest and avoid foods that are high in fibre or difficult to swallow.

Recipes:

1. Avocado Smoothie:

Ingredients:
- 1 ripe avocado
- 1 banana
- 1 cup almond milk (unsweetened)
- 1 tablespoon honey (optional)
- 1 tablespoon chia seeds (optional)
- Ice (optional)
- Lemon juice (optional)
- Water (optional)

Instructions:
1. Halve the avocado and remove the pit. Place the flesh in a blender after scooping it out.
2. Add the banana, almond milk, honey (if desired), chia seeds (if desired), ice (if desired), lemon juice

(if desired), and water (if desired). Blend until smooth. Enjoy immediately!

Nutritional Information: This smoothie is rich in healthy fats from the avocado, carbohydrates from the banana, protein from the chia seeds (if desired), and calcium from the almond milk (unsweetened). It's also high in calories due to the avocado and honey (if desired). This smoothie is an excellent source of nutrition for managing weight loss during leukaemia treatment. Optional ingredients such as ice and lemon juice can be added for personal preference. This recipe serves one person but can easily be doubled or tripled for multiple servings. Refrigerate any leftovers in an airtight container for up to 24 hours. Reheat in the microwave or on the stovetop before consuming again.

2. Quinoa Salad:

Ingredients:
- 1 cup cooked quinoa (rinsed)
- 1 cup cherry tomatoes (halved)
- 1 cup cucumber (diced)
- 1 cup red bell pepper (diced)
- 1/2 cup red onion (diced)
- 1/4 cup parsley (chopped)
- 2 tablespoons olive oil (extra virgin)
- 2 tablespoons lemon juice (freshly squeezed)
- Salt (to taste)
- Pepper (to taste)

Instructions:
1. Rinse the quinoa under cold water using a fine mesh strainer or cheesecloth until the water runs clear. Cook according to package instructions until fluffy and set aside to cool completely before adding other ingredients.
2. In a large mixing bowl, combine the cooked quinoa, cherry tomatoes, cucumber, red bell pepper, red onion, and parsley. Mix well until all ingredients are evenly distributed throughout the salad.
3. Drizzle olive oil and lemon juice over the salad mixture and season with salt and pepper to taste. Toss gently until all ingredients are coated with dressing evenly before serving immediately!
Nutritional Information: This salad is rich in complex carbohydrates from the quinoa, vitamins C and K from the cherry tomatoes, cucumber, red bell pepper, vitamin A from the parsley, healthy fats from the olive oil, and lemon juice adds flavour without adding calories! This recipe serves four people but can easily be doubled or tripled for multiple servings depending on your needs! Refrigerate any leftovers in an airtight container for up to three days!
Reheat in the microwave or on the stovetop before consuming again!

Conclusion: In conclusion, maintaining a healthy diet during leukaemia treatment is crucial for managing side effects such as nausea, fatigue, and weight loss while supporting healing processes within your body! By following our recipes provided above along with our tips for managing side effects through dietary choices you can make sure you get all necessary nutrients while still enjoying delicious meals! Remember to always consult with your healthcare provider before making any significant changes to your dietary habits while undergoing cancer treatments!

How This CookBook can Help

The Leukaemia Diet cookbook is a unique resource for individuals undergoing treatment for leukaemia. This cookbook is designed to provide nutritional guidance and delicious recipe ideas that can help support the body during this challenging time.

Leukaemia is a blood malignancy that affects the bone marrow. Treatment for leukaemia can be intense and may include chemotherapy, radiation therapy, or stem cell transplantation. These treatments can take a toll on the body, causing side effects such as fatigue, nausea, and loss of appetite.

The Leukaemia Diet cookbook recognizes the importance of maintaining a healthy diet during treatment. The cookbook provides information on the nutritional needs of individuals with leukaemia, as well as tips for managing common side effects of treatment.

The recipes in this cookbook are specifically designed to meet the nutritional needs of individuals with leukaemia. They are low in fat and salt, and high in protein, fibre, and other essential nutrients. Many of the recipes also incorporate ingredients that have been shown to have anti-inflammatory properties, which can help support the body during treatment.

Some examples of recipes from the Leukaemia Diet cookbook include:

- Grilled chicken with roasted vegetables: This dish is packed with protein and fibre, and the grilled chicken provides essential amino acids that are important for building and repairing cells.
- Quinoa salad with avocado and cherry tomatoes: Quinoa is a great source of protein and fibre, while avocado provides healthy fats that can help combat fatigue.
- Lentil soup with kale: Lentils are a good source of protein and fibre, while kale is rich in iron and other essential nutrients that can help support the body during treatment.

In addition to providing nutritional guidance and recipe ideas, the Leukaemia Diet cookbook also includes tips for managing common side effects of treatment. For example, it provides suggestions for managing nausea by incorporating ginger into recipes or serving small, frequent meals throughout the day. It also provides tips for managing fatigue by suggesting simple, easy-to-prepare meals that require minimal effort.

Overall, the Leukaemia Diet cookbook is an invaluable resource for individuals undergoing treatment for leukaemia. By providing nutritional guidance and delicious recipe ideas, this cookbook can help support the body during treatment and promote overall health and wellbeing.

CHAPTER ONE

Building a Nutrient-Rich Foundation

Key Nutrients for Leukaemia Patients

Leukaemia is a type of cancer that affects the blood and bone marrow, causing a decrease in healthy blood cells and an increase in abnormal white blood cells. Proper nutrition is crucial for leukaemia patients as it helps to maintain a healthy weight, manage symptoms, and support the body's immune system during treatment. Here are some key nutrients that leukaemia patients should focus on to build a nutrient-rich foundation:

- Protein: Protein is essential for building and repairing cells, including those affected by leukaemia. Leukaemia patients may experience muscle wasting due to the disease or treatment, making it important to consume enough protein to maintain muscle mass. Good sources of protein include lean meats, poultry, fish, beans, and lentils.

- Iron: Iron is necessary for the production of red blood cells, which are often affected by leukaemia. Patients may experience anaemia due to a lack of red blood cells, making it important to consume foods rich in iron. Iron-rich foods include red meat, chicken, beans, and fortified cereals.

- Folate: Folate is important for the production of red blood cells and helps to prevent anaemia. Leukaemia patients may be prescribed folic acid supplements to help prevent anaemia caused by chemotherapy or radiation therapy. Leafy green vegetables, citrus fruits, and fortified cereals are all high in folate.

- Calcium: Calcium is important for maintaining bone health, which can be affected by leukaemia treatment. Patients may experience osteoporosis or bone fractures due to treatment-induced bone loss. Calcium-rich foods include dairy products, leafy green vegetables, and fortified cereals.

- Vitamin D: Vitamin D is necessary for the absorption of calcium and helps to maintain bone health. Leukaemia patients may be at risk for vitamin D deficiency due to decreased sunlight exposure during treatment. Good sources of vitamin D include fatty fish, fortified cereals, and sunlight exposure (with sunscreen).

- Fibre: Fibre is important for maintaining bowel regularity, which can be affected by leukaemia treatment. Patients may experience constipation due to treatment-induced dehydration or medication side effects. Good sources of fibre include whole grains, fruits, and vegetables.

- Hydration: Hydration is crucial for maintaining fluid balance in the body and preventing dehydration during treatment-induced nausea or vomiting. Patients should aim to drink at least eight glasses of water per day and avoid sugary drinks that can lead to dehydration due to increased urination.

In conclusion, leukaemia patients should focus on consuming a variety of nutrient-rich foods to support their health during treatment. A registered dietitian can provide personalised nutrition guidance based on individual needs and preferences.

Incorporating Essential Vitamins and Minerals

Building a nutrient-rich foundation for your body is essential for maintaining optimal health and preventing chronic diseases. While a balanced diet can provide most of the essential vitamins and minerals, some individuals may require supplements to meet their daily requirements. In this article, we will discuss some of the most important vitamins and minerals and how to incorporate them into your diet.

Vitamin D

Vitamin D is necessary for strong bones because it aids in calcium absorption. It also plays a role in immune system function and reducing inflammation. The best source of vitamin D is sunlight, but it can also be found in fatty fish, eggs, and fortified foods such as milk and cereal. For individuals who do not get enough sunlight or consume these foods regularly, a supplement may be necessary.

Calcium

Calcium is essential for the formation and maintenance of strong bones and teeth. It can be found in dairy products such as milk, yoghurt, and cheese, as well as leafy green vegetables like kale and spinach. For individuals who are lactose intolerant or do not consume dairy products, calcium supplements may be necessary.

Iron

Iron is required for the formation of red blood cells, which transport oxygen throughout the body. It can be found in meat, poultry, seafood, beans, and fortified cereals. For vegetarians or individuals with low iron levels, a supplement may be necessary. However, it is important to note that excessive iron intake can lead to health problems such as constipation and increased risk of cancer.

Magnesium

Magnesium is involved in over 300 enzymatic reactions in the body and is essential for bone health, muscle function, and nerve function. Leafy green vegetables, nuts, seeds, and whole grains all contain it. Magnesium supplements may be necessary for individuals with low magnesium levels or those who have difficulty consuming enough through diet alone.

Vitamin B12

Vitamin B12 is required for nerve function and red blood cell formation. It is primarily found in animal products such as meat, poultry, and dairy products. For vegetarians or individuals who follow a vegan diet, a supplement may be necessary to prevent deficiency.

Incorporating these vitamins and minerals into your diet can be achieved through a variety of foods and supplements. Here are some tips:

1. Eat a variety of foods from all food groups to ensure you are getting a wide range of nutrients.

2. Choose whole foods over processed foods whenever possible to ensure you are getting all the necessary nutrients without added sugars or preservatives.

3. Incorporate fortified foods into your diet to increase your intake of certain vitamins and minerals that may be lacking in your diet due to dietary restrictions or preferences.

4. Consult with a healthcare provider or registered dietitian to determine if supplements are necessary based on your individual needs and any underlying medical conditions.

5. Be aware of potential interactions between supplements and medications you may be taking to avoid any negative side effects or interactions that could compromise your health.

Tips for Meal Planning and Preparation

Meal planning and preparation are crucial components of building a nutrient-rich foundation for a healthy lifestyle. Here are some pointers to get you started:

1. Understand your nutritional needs:

Before you start meal planning, it's essential to understand your nutritional needs. This will help you create a meal plan that provides all the necessary nutrients your body needs. Consult a registered dietitian or nutritionist to determine your daily calorie intake, macronutrient ratios, and micronutrient requirements.

2. Plan ahead:

Set aside some time each week to plan your meals. This will help you stay organised, save time, and ensure that you have all the necessary ingredients on hand. Consider planning meals for the entire week or month to make it easier to stick to your plan.

3. Focus on whole foods:

Choose whole foods as the foundation of your meals. Fruits, vegetables, whole grains, lean meats, and healthy fats are examples of these. Avoid processed foods as much as possible as they often contain added sugars, salt, and unhealthy fats.

Eating a variety of foods will ensure that you're getting all the necessary nutrients your body needs. Aim to include a variety of colours on your plate to ensure that you're getting a range of vitamins and minerals.

Spend some time each week prepping your meals in advance. This will make it easier to stick to your meal plan during the week and save time during busy days. Consider prepping ingredients like chopped vegetables, cooked grains, and marinated proteins to make meal assembly quick and easy.

It's essential to practise portion control to ensure that you're consuming the right amount of calories for your body's needs. Use measuring cups and food scales to ensure that you're eating appropriate portions of each food group.

Eating a nutrient-rich diet doesn't have to be boring! Experiment with different flavours and spices to make your meals more interesting and enjoyable.

This will help you stick to your meal plan and make healthy eating a sustainable lifestyle choice.

8. Stay hydrated:

Drinking enough water is essential for overall health and wellbeing. Aim to drink at least eight glasses of water per day, more if you're physically active or live in a hot climate.

9. Don't forget about snacks:

Incorporate healthy snacks into your meal plan to help you stay satisfied between meals. Choose snacks that are high in protein and fibre, such as nuts, seeds, Greek yoghourt, or fresh fruit with nut butter.

10. Be flexible:

Remember that meal planning is a guide, not a strict rulebook! Allow yourself some flexibility in your meal plan to accommodate unexpected events or changes in appetite. The goal is to build a sustainable lifestyle that works for you in the long term.

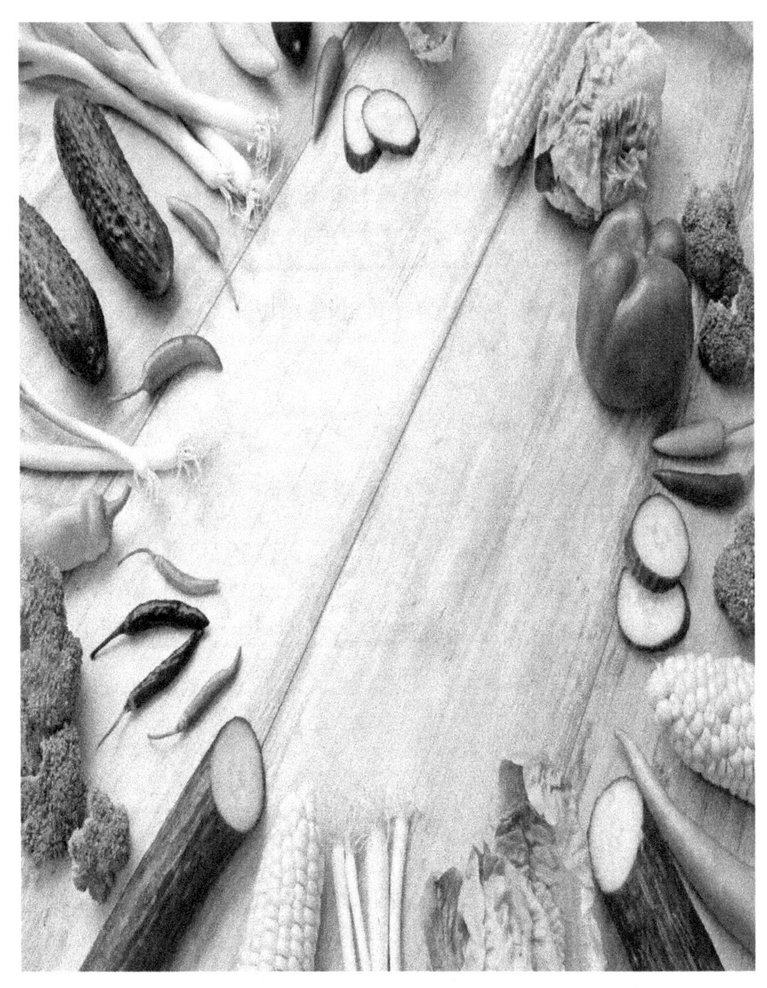

CHAPTER TWO

Recipes for Energy and Strength

High-Protein Dishes for Endurance

When undergoing treatment for leukaemia, it's essential to maintain a healthy and balanced diet that provides the necessary nutrients to support your body's needs. Protein is a crucial component of this diet, as it helps build and repair tissues, including muscle mass, which is essential for endurance during treatment. Here are some high-protein dishes that are perfect for maintaining energy and strength during leukaemia treatment:

- Grilled Chicken and Vegetable Skewers

Ingredients:
- 4 boneless, skinless chicken breasts, cut into cubes
- 2 bell peppers, cut into chunks
- 1 red onion, cut into chunks
- 1 zucchini, cut into rounds
- 1 yellow squash, cut into rounds
- 2 tbsp olive oil
- Salt and pepper to taste
- Lemon wedges for serving

Instructions:
1. Preheat the grill to medium-high heat.

2. Thread chicken and vegetables onto skewers alternately.

3. Season the skewers with salt and pepper after brushing them with olive oil.

4. Grill skewers for 8-10 minutes on each side or until chicken is cooked through.

5. Serve with lemon wedges.

Nutritional Information (per serving): Calories: 300, Protein: 30g, Carbohydrates: 15g, Fat: 13g, Fibre: 3g, Sugar: 8g

- Quinoa Salad with Grilled Shrimp and Avocado Dressing

Ingredients:
- 1 cup quinoa, rinsed and drained
- 2 cups low-sodium chicken broth
- 1 pound large peeled and deveined shrimp
- Salt and pepper to taste
- 2 tbsp olive oil, divided
- 1 avocado, pitted and peeled
- Juice of 1 lime
- 1 garlic clove, minced
- Handful of fresh cilantro leaves, chopped
- Salt and pepper to taste (optional)
- Cherry tomatoes and cucumber slices for garnish (optional)

Instructions:
1. In a medium saucepan, combine quinoa and chicken broth. Bring to a boil over high heat.

Reduce heat to low and simmer until quinoa is tender and liquid is absorbed, about 15 minutes. Fluff with a fork and set aside.

2. Preheat the grill to medium-high heat. Season shrimp with salt and pepper. Brush with olive oil and grill for 2-3 minutes on each side or until pink and cooked through. Set aside.

3. In a blender or food processor, combine avocado, lime juice, garlic, cilantro leaves, salt, and pepper (optional). Blend until smooth. Add remaining olive oil while blending until desired consistency is reached. Set aside.

4. In a large bowl, combine cooked quinoa and grilled shrimp. Pour avocado dressing over the top and toss to combine. Garnish with cherry tomatoes and cucumber slices (optional). Serve immediately.

Nutritional Information (per serving): Calories: 370, Protein: 28g, Carbohydrates: 36g, Fat: 16g, Fibre: 7g, Sugar: 2g

- Turkey Chili with Brown Rice and Avocado Salsa (Vegan Option Available)

Ingredients (Turkey Chilli):
- 1 lb ground turkey breast (or plant-based meat substitute)
- 1 onion, chopped
- 2 garlic cloves, minced
- 2 bell peppers (any colour), chopped
- 1 can (28 oz) crushed tomatoes (no salt added)

- 2 cans (15 oz each) kidney beans (no salt added),
drained and rinsed well
- 2 tbsp chilli powder (adjust to taste)
- Salt and pepper to taste (optional)
- Fresh parsley or cilantro leaves for garnish
(optional)

Instructions: (Turkey Chilli)
1. In a large pot or Dutch oven over medium heat,
cook ground turkey breast until browned. Remove
from the pot using a slotted spoon and set aside on
a plate lined with paper towels to drain excess fat.
2. In the same pot over medium heat, sauté onion
until softened (about 5 minutes).
Add garlic and bell peppers; cook for another
minute or until fragrant.
3. Add crushed tomatoes, cooked turkey breast (or
plant-based meat substitute), kidney beans
(drained), chilli powder (adjust to taste), salt
(optional), and pepper (optional).
Stir well to combine all ingredients evenly in the
pot/Dutch oven; bring chilli to a boil over high heat;
then reduce heat to low; cover pot/Dutch oven;
simmer chilli for about 20 minutes or until heated
through; stir occasionally during cooking process;
adjust seasoning as needed before serving hot with
brown rice; garnish with fresh parsley or cilantro
leaves if desired before serving hot; serve
immediately with avocado salsa on the side (see
below).

Nutritional Information (per serving): Calories: 340 (with ground turkey breast); Calories: 260 (with plant-based meat substitute); Protein: 34g (with ground turkey breast); Protein: 24g (with plant-based meat substitute); Carbohydrates:

Energy-Boosting Smoothies and Snacks

When undergoing treatment for leukaemia, it's essential to maintain a healthy and balanced diet that provides the necessary nutrients to support your body's needs. In addition to traditional meals, incorporating energy-boosting smoothies and snacks into your diet can provide a quick and convenient source of fuel to help you power through your day. Here are some delicious and nutritious recipes to try:

1. Green Goddess Smoothie
Ingredients:
- 1 banana
- 1 cup spinach
- 1 cup kale
- 1 cup almond milk
- 1/2 avocado
- 1 tbsp honey
- 1 tbsp chia seeds
- 1 tbsp flaxseeds
- 1 cup ice cubes

Instructions:
Blend all ingredients in a blender until smooth. Pour into a glass and serve right away.

2. Berry Blast Smoothie
Ingredients:
- 1 cup mixed berries (fresh or frozen)
- 1 banana
- 1 cup almond milk
- 1 tbsp honey
- 1 tbsp chia seeds
- 1 tbsp flaxseeds
- 1 cup ice cubes

Instructions:
Blend all ingredients in a blender until smooth. Pour into a glass and serve right away.

3. Apple Cinnamon Energy Bites
Ingredients:
- 2 medium apples, peeled and grated
- 1/2 cup rolled oats
- 1/4 cup almond butter
- 2 tbsp honey
- 2 tbsp chia seeds
- 2 tbsp flaxseeds
- 1 tsp ground cinnamon
- Pinch of salt

Instructions:
Combine all ingredients in a mixing basin and thoroughly combine. Roll the mixture into small

balls and refrigerate for at least an hour before serving. These bites can be stored in the fridge for up to a week.

4. Banana Oat Bars (Gluten-Free)
Ingredients:
For the bars:
- 3 ripe bananas, mashed (about 3 cups)
- 3 cups rolled oats (use gluten-free oats if necessary)
- 1/2 cup almond butter (or your favourite nut butter)
- 1/4 cup honey (or maple syrup if vegan)
- 2 tbsp chia seeds (optional)
- Pinch of salt (optional)

For the coating:
- 1/4 cup unsweetened shredded coconut (optional)
- 2 tbsp honey (or maple syrup for a vegan option) (optional)

Instructions:
Preheat the oven to 350°F (180°C).
Grease an 8x8 inch baking dish with cooking spray or line it with parchment paper. In a mixing bowl, combine mashed bananas, rolled oats, almond butter, honey, chia seeds, and salt (if using). Mix until all of the ingredients are uniformly distributed. Spread the ingredients out evenly in the prepared baking dish. Bake for about 25 minutes, or until the top is golden brown. Let it cool in the pan for about ten minutes before removing it from

the pan and slicing it into bars. For the coating, mix shredded coconut and honey in a small mixing bowl until well combined. Spread the coating on top of each bar before serving. These bars can be stored in an airtight container in the fridge for up to a week or frozen for up to three months. These energy bites and bars are packed with nutrients that will provide you with sustained energy throughout the day. They're also easy to prepare and can be made ahead of time for convenience. Incorporating these recipes into your diet can help you maintain your energy levels during leukaemia treatment while also providing your body with essential nutrients it needs to stay healthy and strong.

CHAPTER THREE

Immune-Boosting Delights

Foods to Support the Immune System

Leukaemia is a type of cancer that affects the blood and bone marrow, leading to a weakened immune system. Eating a healthy and balanced diet can help support the immune system and provide the body with the necessary nutrients to fight off infections. In this cookbook, we will be sharing immune-boosting delights that are not only delicious but also packed with nutrients that support the immune system.

☐ Citrus Salad

Citrus fruits such as oranges, lemons, and limes are rich in vitamin C, which is essential for a healthy immune system. This citrus salad is a refreshing and healthy way to start your day.

Ingredients:
- 2 oranges, peeled and segmented
- 2 grapefruits, peeled and segmented
- 1 lemon, peeled and segmented
- 1 lime, peeled and segmented
- 1 tbsp honey
- 1 tbsp olive oil
- Salt and pepper to taste

Instructions:
1. In a large bowl, combine the oranges, grapefruits, lemon, and lime segments.
2. Drizzle honey and olive oil over the fruit.
3. Season with salt and pepper to taste.
4. Toss gently to combine all ingredients.
5. Serve chilled.

☐ Turmeric Ginger Tea

Turmeric and ginger are both anti-inflammatory spices that have been shown to boost the immune system. This tea is a warming and comforting drink that is perfect for chilly evenings.

Ingredients:
- 1 inch peeled and grated fresh ginger
- 1 tsp turmeric powder
- 4 cups water
- Honey (optional) to taste
- Lemon wedges (optional) for garnish

Instructions:
1. Bring water to a boil in a medium saucepan.
2. Add ginger and turmeric powder to the boiling water. Reduce heat to low and let it simmer for 5-7 minutes until the water turns yellow in colour.
3. Strain the tea into a teapot or mugs using a fine mesh strainer or cheesecloth to remove any solids. Discard the solids.

4. Add honey to taste (optional). Stir well until honey is dissolved completely.
5. Garnish with lemon wedges (optional). Serve hot.

☐ Berry Smoothie Bowl

Berries such as strawberries, blueberries, raspberries, and blackberries are rich in antioxidants that help boost the immune system. This smoothie bowl is a healthy breakfast option that is both delicious and nutritious.

Ingredients:
For the smoothie:
- 1 cup mixed berries (fresh or frozen)
- 1 banana (frozen)
- 1 cup almond milk (unsweetened)
- 1 tbsp honey (optional) to taste for sweetness (use maple syrup for vegan option)
- 1 tsp chia seeds (optional) for added texture and nutrition (use flaxseeds for vegan option)
- Ice cubes (optional) if desired for thicker consistency or colder temperature preference (use frozen berries instead of ice cubes for vegan option) For the toppings:
- Fresh berries (strawberries, blueberries, raspberries, blackberries) for garnish and added nutrition value (use any berries you prefer or have on hand) - Granola for added crunchiness (use gluten-free granola if preferred) - Almond slices or other nuts/seeds of choice for added protein and

healthy fats (use any nuts/seeds you prefer or have on hand) - Coconut flakes for added texture (use unsweetened coconut flakes if preferred)

Instructions:
1. In a blender, combine mixed berries, frozen banana, almond milk, honey (optional), chia seeds (optional), and ice cubes (optional). Blend until the mixture is smooth and creamy.
2. Pour the smoothie into a bowl.
3. Top with fresh berries, granola, almond slices/nuts/seeds of choice, and coconut flakes as desired for added texture and nutrition value. Serve immediately as a refreshing breakfast option or snack alternative that's packed with nutrients! We hope you enjoy these immune-boosting delights! Remember to always consult with your healthcare provider before making any significant dietary changes, especially if you have leukaemia or any other medical condition that requires dietary restrictions or modifications based on your specific needs and preferences!

Recipes Packed with Antioxidants

Leukaemia is a blood malignancy that affects the bone marrow. It weakens the immune system, making it difficult for the body to fight off infections and diseases. A healthy diet rich in antioxidants can help boost the immune system and aid in the recovery process for leukaemia patients. In this cookbook, we will provide recipes packed with antioxidants that are not only delicious but also beneficial for immune-boosting delights.

1. Berry Blast Smoothie Bowl

Ingredients:
- 1 cup mixed berries (fresh or frozen)
- 1 banana
- 1 cup almond milk
- 1 tbsp chia seeds
- 1 tbsp honey (optional)
- 1/4 cup granola
- 1/4 cup sliced almonds
- 1/4 cup blueberries (for garnish)

Instructions:
1. Blend mixed berries, banana, almond milk, chia seeds, and honey (if using) until smooth.
2. Pour the smoothie into a bowl.
3. Top with granola, sliced almonds, and blueberries.
4. Serve immediately and enjoy!

Benefits:
Berries are rich in antioxidants such as vitamin C and anthocyanins, which help boost the immune system. Chia seeds are a great source of omega-3 fatty acids, fibre, and protein, which also aid in immune function. Almonds are high in vitamin E, another antioxidant that helps protect cells from damage.

Ingredients:
- 2 cups kale (chopped)
- 1 cup quinoa (cooked)
- 1 red bell pepper (chopped)
- 1 yellow bell pepper (chopped)
- 1 zucchini (chopped)
- 1 red onion (chopped)
- 2 tbsp olive oil
- 2 tbsp balsamic vinegar
- Salt and pepper to taste
- Feta cheese (optional)
- Lemon wedges (for garnish)

Instructions:
1. Preheat the oven to 400°F (200°C). Line a baking sheet with parchment paper.
2. Toss chopped bell peppers, zucchini, and red onion with olive oil, salt, and pepper. Spread them out on the baking sheet that has been prepared. Roast for 20-25 minutes or until vegetables are tender and lightly browned. Set aside to cool slightly.
3. In a large bowl, combine chopped kale and cooked quinoa. Add roasted vegetables and toss gently to combine. Drizzle with balsamic vinegar and toss again to distribute evenly.
Top with feta cheese (if using). Serve with lemon wedges on the side for squeezing over the salad before eating. Enjoy!

Benefits:
Kale is an excellent source of vitamin C, vitamin K, and beta-carotene, all of which are powerful antioxidants that help boost the immune system. Quinoa is high in protein and fibre, which also aid in immune function.
Bell peppers are rich in vitamin C, while zucchini is a good source of vitamin A and potassium.
Feta cheese adds a tangy flavour to the salad while also providing calcium and protein. Balsamic vinegar is a good source of antioxidants called polyphenols that help protect cells from damage. Lemon adds a refreshing citrus flavour while also providing vitamin C.
Overall, this salad is packed with antioxidants that help boost the immune system while also being delicious!

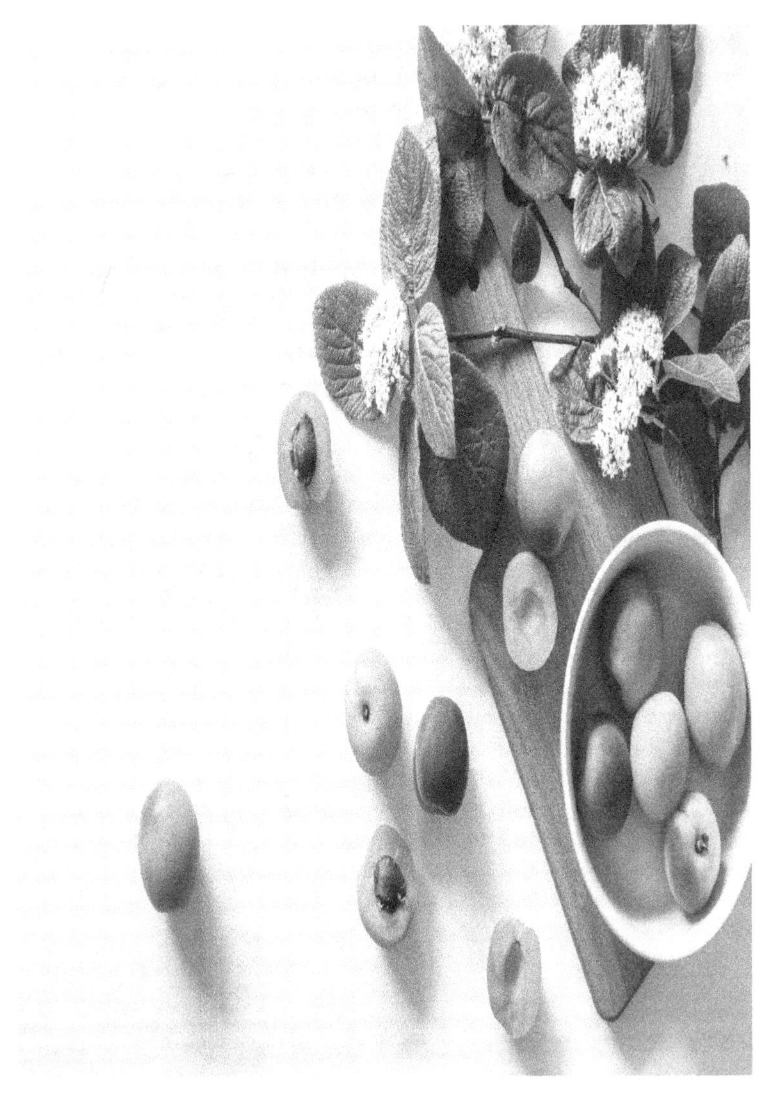

CHAPTER FOUR

Easy-to-Digest Comfort Foods

Gentle on the Stomach Recipes

When dealing with leukaemia, a cancer of the blood cells, it's essential to follow a diet that is gentle on the stomach and helps support the body's immune system. These recipes are designed to be easy-to-digest comfort foods that will provide nourishment and support during this challenging time.

1. Chicken and Vegetable Soup

Ingredients:
- 1 lb boneless, skinless chicken breasts, cubed
- 1 onion, chopped
- 2 cloves garlic, minced
- 2 carrots, peeled and chopped
- 2 celery stalks, chopped
- 1 zucchini, chopped
- 1 can (14 oz) low-sodium chicken broth
- 1 can (14 oz) low-sodium vegetable broth
- 1 tbsp olive oil
- Salt and pepper to taste

Instructions:

1. In a large pot over medium heat, heat the olive oil. Cook until the chicken is browned on all sides. Set aside after removing from the saucepan.
2. Add onion, garlic, carrots, celery, and zucchini to the pot. Cook until vegetables are softened.
3. Add chicken broth and vegetable broth to the pot. Bring to a boil, then reduce to a low heat and continue to cook for 10 minutes.
4. Add chicken back to the pot and simmer for an additional 5 minutes. Season with salt and pepper to taste. Serve hot.

2. Baked Apples with Cinnamon and Oats

Ingredients:
- 4 apples, cored and halved
- 1/2 cup rolled oats
- 1/4 cup chopped walnuts
- 2 tbsp brown sugar
- 1 tsp ground cinnamon
- 2 tbsp unsalted butter, melted
- Vanilla ice cream (optional) for serving

Instructions:

1. Preheat the oven to 375°F (190°C). Line a baking sheet with parchment paper.
2. In a bowl, mix together oats, walnuts, brown sugar, cinnamon, and melted butter until well combined. Spoon mixture into apple halves. Place apples on a prepared baking sheet and bake for 25-30 minutes or until the apples are tender and

the filling is golden brown. Serve hot with vanilla ice cream if desired.

3. Ginger Tea with Honey and Lemon

Ingredients:
- 2 inch piece fresh ginger root, peeled and sliced thinly
- 4 cups water
- Juice of 1 lemon
- Honey to taste (optional)

Instructions:
1. In a saucepan, bring water and ginger to a boil over high heat. Reduce heat to low and simmer for 5 minutes or until ginger is fragrant. Remove from heat and let steep for an additional 5 minutes. Strain tea into a mug or pitcher. Stir in lemon juice and honey if desired. Serve hot or cold over ice. Enjoy!

Nourishing Soups and Broths

When undergoing treatment for leukaemia, it's essential to consume nutritious and easy-to-digest foods that can help support the body's immune system and provide essential nutrients. Soups and broths are an excellent choice as they are packed with vitamins, minerals, and protein that can aid in recovery. In this cookbook, we will share some easy-to-digest soup and broth recipes that are perfect for individuals undergoing leukaemia treatment.

1. Chicken and Vegetable Broth

Ingredients:
- 1 whole chicken (skinless)
- 1 onion (quartered)
- 2 carrots (peeled and chopped)
- 2 celery stalks (chopped)
- 1 garlic clove (minced)
- 1 bay leaf
- Salt and pepper to taste
- Water (enough to cover the chicken)

Instructions:
1. Rinse the chicken thoroughly and pat dry with paper towels.
2. In a large pot, add the chicken, onion, carrots, celery, garlic, bay leaf, salt, and pepper.
3. Pour enough water to cover the chicken completely.
4. Bring the pot to a boil over high heat, then reduce the heat to low and let it simmer for 1 hour or until the chicken is cooked through.
5. Remove the chicken from the pot and let it cool before shredding it into small pieces. Discard the bay leaf.
6. Strain the broth through a fine mesh strainer to remove any solids. Discard the solids.

7. Return the strained broth to the pot and add the shredded chicken back in. Reheat over low heat until warm.

8. Serve hot and enjoy!

2. Lemon Ginger Chicken Soup

Ingredients:
- 2 boneless, skinless chicken breasts (cubed)
- 1 onion (chopped)
- 2 garlic cloves (minced)
- 2 inch piece of ginger (peeled and grated)
- 4 cups chicken broth (low sodium)
- Juice of 1 lemon
- Salt and pepper to taste
- Fresh parsley (chopped for garnish)
- Water (enough to cover the chicken)

Instructions:
1. In a large pot, add the chicken, onion, garlic, ginger, salt, pepper, lemon juice, and enough water to cover the chicken completely. Bring to a boil over high heat then reduce heat to low and let it simmer for 20 minutes or until the chicken is cooked through.
2. Add the low sodium chicken broth to the pot and let it simmer for an additional 10 minutes or until heated through. Taste and adjust seasoning as needed. Garnish with fresh parsley before serving hot. Enjoy!
3. Vegetable Miso Soup (Gluten-Free Option Available)

Ingredients: (Gluten-Free Option Available)
For Gluten-Free Option: Use gluten-free miso paste instead of regular miso paste which contains wheat or barley as a thickener or flavouring agent in some brands of miso paste.
Check your miso paste label carefully for gluten content before purchasing or using it in this recipe!
- 4 cups of vegetable broth (low sodium) - 1 onion (chopped)
- 2 garlic cloves (minced)
- 2 inch piece of ginger (peeled and grated)
- 4 cups of mixed vegetables (carrots, celery, mushrooms, snow peas, bok choy or any other vegetables you prefer)
- Salt and pepper to taste
- Miso paste (to taste)
- Fresh parsley (chopped for garnish)

Instructions:
1. In a large pot, add vegetable broth, onion, garlic, ginger, salt, pepper, mixed vegetables, and bring it to a boil over high heat then reduce heat to low and let it simmer for 20 minutes or until vegetables are tender but not mushy!
2. Add miso paste to taste while stirring constantly until dissolved completely in soup broth!
Taste soup broth again for seasoning adjustment if necessary before serving hot with fresh parsley as garnish!
Enjoy your nourishing soups and broths!

These recipes are packed with essential nutrients that can help support your body during leukaemia treatment while being gentle on your digestive system at the same time! Remember always to check with your healthcare provider before making any significant dietary changes or trying new recipes during your treatment!

ANTI-NAUSEA SMOOTHIE

@juna.moms

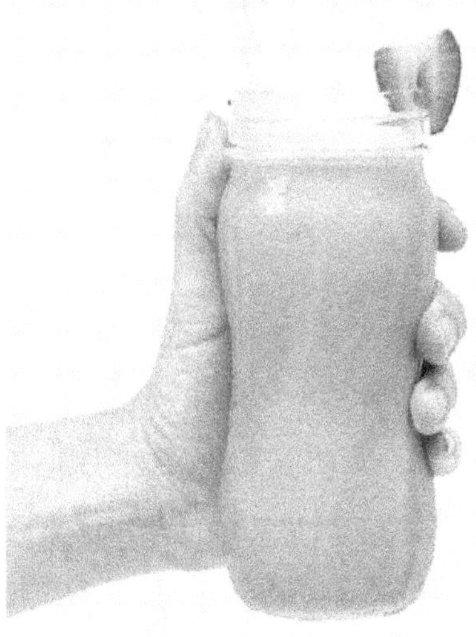

1 banana

7 strawberries

1/2 tsp fresh ginger

1/2 cup coconut milk

1/4 cup rolled oats

1/2 teaspoon vanilla, optional

ice/water to taste

Add all ingredients to blender. Blend for 30-60 seconds.

CHAPTER FIVE

Managing Side Effects Through Nutrition

Alleviating Nausea with Thoughtful Food Choices

Leukaemia is a blood malignancy that affects the bone marrow. One of the most common side effects of leukaemia treatment is nausea, which can make it challenging for patients to eat and maintain a healthy weight. However, making thoughtful food choices can help alleviate nausea and support overall health during treatment.

Here are some nutrition tips for managing nausea during leukaemia treatment:

- Eat small, frequent meals: Eating smaller, more frequent meals throughout the day can help prevent nausea by keeping the stomach from becoming too full. This also allows the body to absorb nutrients more efficiently.

- Choose foods that are easy to digest: During treatment, the digestive system may be compromised, making it difficult to digest certain foods. Choosing foods that are easy to digest, such as cooked vegetables, fruits, and whole-grain breads, can help prevent nausea and discomfort.

- Avoid spicy and fatty foods: Spicy and fatty foods can irritate the stomach and exacerbate nausea. Instead, choose mild-flavoured foods that are low in fat and spice.

- Stay hydrated: Dehydration can worsen nausea, so it's essential to drink plenty of fluids throughout the day. Water, herbal tea, and clear broths are good choices.

- Incorporate protein: Protein is essential for building and repairing tissues in the body. Choosing protein-rich foods such as chicken, fish, beans, and tofu can help maintain muscle mass during treatment.

- Limit caffeine and alcohol: Caffeine and alcohol can both worsen nausea, so it's best to limit or avoid these beverages during treatment.

- Consult a registered dietitian: A registered dietitian can provide personalised nutrition advice based on individual needs and preferences during leukaemia treatment. They can also offer strategies for managing specific side effects such as taste changes or mouth sores.

In summary, making thoughtful food choices can help alleviate nausea during leukaemia treatment by choosing small, frequent meals, easy-to-digest foods, staying hydrated, incorporating protein, limiting caffeine and alcohol, and consulting a registered dietitian for personalised advice. By following these tips, patients can maintain a healthy weight and support overall health during treatment.

Addressing Taste Changes with Flavourful Recipes

When undergoing treatment for leukaemia, patients may experience a range of side effects that can affect their sense of taste. Chemotherapy and radiation therapy can cause changes in taste, making certain foods taste different or less appealing. This can lead to a decrease in appetite and difficulty meeting nutritional needs. In this cookbook, we will provide flavourful recipes that are designed to address taste changes and help manage side effects through nutrition.

1. Spicy Ginger Chicken Stir-Fry

Ingredients:
- 1 lb boneless, skinless chicken breast, cut into thin strips
- 1 tbsp olive oil

- 1 onion, chopped
- 2 garlic cloves, minced
- 1 tbsp grated fresh ginger
- 1 red bell pepper, sliced
- 1 green bell pepper, sliced
- 2 cups broccoli florets
- 2 tbsp soy sauce
- 1 tbsp honey
- 1 tbsp rice vinegar
- 1 tsp red pepper flakes (adjust to taste)
- Salt and pepper to taste

Instructions:
1. In a large skillet over medium-high heat, heat the olive oil. Cook until the chicken is browned on all sides, about 5 minutes. Set aside after removing from the skillet.
2. Add onion, garlic, and ginger to the skillet and cook until softened, about 3 minutes. Add bell peppers and broccoli and cook until vegetables are tender, about 5 minutes.
3. Add chicken back to the skillet. In a small bowl, whisk together soy sauce, honey, rice vinegar, and red pepper flakes. Pour over the chicken and vegetables and stir until everything is coated in the sauce. Season with salt and pepper to taste. Serve hot over rice or noodles.

This dish is packed with protein from the chicken and vegetables that are rich in vitamins and minerals. The spicy ginger flavour can help stimulate appetite and improve taste perception for those experiencing changes in taste due to treatment.

2. Sweet Potato Black Bean Chilli

Ingredients:
- 2 tbsp olive oil
- 1 onion, chopped
- 3 garlic cloves, minced
- 2 sweet potatoes, peeled and diced
- 2 cans drained and rinsed black beans
- 1 can (undrained) chopped tomatoes with green chiles
- 4 cups vegetable broth
- 2 tbsp chilli powder (adjust to taste)
- Salt and pepper to taste
- Optional toppings: avocado, sour cream, cilantro, lime wedges

Instructions:
1. In a large pot over medium heat, heat the olive oil. Cook until the onion and garlic are softened, about 3 minutes. Add sweet potatoes and cook until slightly softened, about 5 minutes.
2. Add black beans, diced tomatoes with green chilies (undrained), vegetable broth, chilli powder, salt, and pepper to the pot. Stir Everything together and bring to a simmer. Cook for 20 minutes, or until sweet potatoes are cooked. Serve hot with desired toppings.

This chilli is rich in fibre from the sweet potatoes and black beans as well as vitamins A and C from the sweet potatoes. The spicy chilli powder can help stimulate appetite and improve taste perception for those experiencing changes in taste due to treatment. The acidity from the tomatoes can also help combat mouth sores that may be a side effect of treatment.

3. Lemon Garlic Shrimp Pasta with Spinach Salad Dressing (Gluten-Free)

Ingredients: (For Pasta)
- 8 oz gluten-free spaghetti or linguine (such as brown rice or quinoa pasta)
- 1 pound large peeled and deveined shrimp
- 4 tbsp butter
- 4 garlic cloves, minced
- Juice of 1 lemon
- Salt and pepper to taste (For Salad Dressing)
- 2 cups fresh spinach leaves
- 1/4 cup plain Greek yoghurt
- Juice of half a lemon
- Salt and pepper to taste

Instructions: (For Pasta)
- Cook pasta until al dente according to package directions. Drain pasta and set aside.
- In a large skillet over medium heat, melt butter. Add shrimp and garlic and cook until shrimp are pink on both sides, about 3 minutes per side.

- Add lemon juice to the skillet and stir to combine with the shrimp mixture. Season with salt and pepper to taste. Toss cooked pasta with the shrimp mixture until everything is coated in the sauce. Serve hot with spinach salad dressing on the side for dipping pasta into or drizzling over top of the pasta dish for added flavour (optional). (For Salad Dressing)
- In a blender or food processor, combine spinach leaves, Greek yoghurt, lemon juice, salt, and pepper until smooth dressing forms (you may need to scrape down sides of blender/processor occasionally).
This dish is rich in protein from the shrimp as well as vitamins A and C from the spinach leaves used in the dressing recipe. The lemon garlic flavour can help stimulate appetite for those experiencing changes in taste due to treatment while also providing a tangy flavour that may help combat mouth sores that may be a side effect of treatment when used as a dressing for the pasta dish instead of being consumed separately as a salad dressing on the side (optional).

These recipes are designed to address taste changes while also providing nutritional benefits that are important for managing side effects during leukaemia treatment such as protein deficiency due to decreased appetite or malnutrition caused by difficulty eating certain foods due to changes in taste perception or mouth sores that may be present during treatment. We hope you find these recipes helpful!

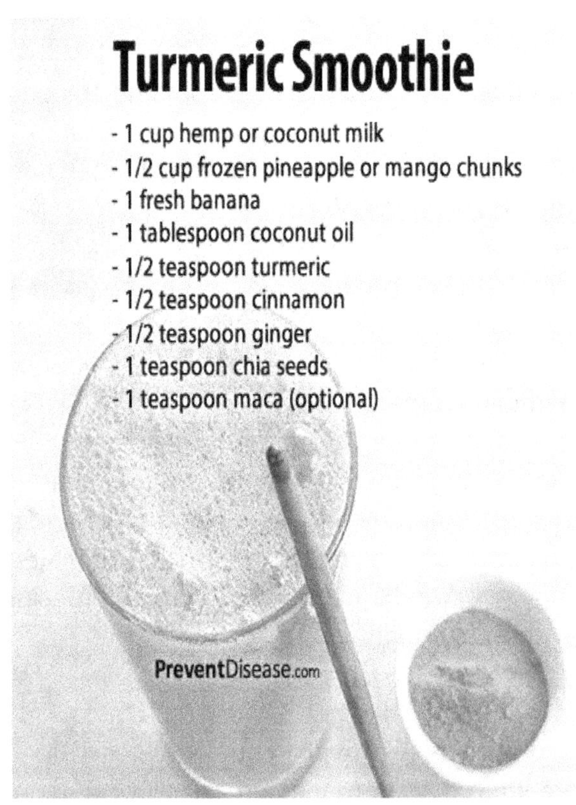

CHAPTER SIX

Mindful Meal Planning

Balancing Macronutrients in Every Meal

Balancing macronutrients in every meal is crucial for individuals undergoing treatment for leukaemia as it helps to maintain a healthy weight, provide essential nutrients, and manage symptoms such as fatigue and nausea. Mindful meal planning involves creating a meal plan that meets the specific nutritional needs of the individual while also considering their preferences, lifestyle, and any dietary restrictions. Here's how to balance macronutrients in every meal for a leukaemia diet cookbook:

1. Understand the role of macronutrients:

Macronutrients are the three main nutrients that provide energy to the body: carbohydrates, proteins, and fats. Each macronutrient serves a distinct function in the body:

- Carbohydrates: Provide energy for the body and brain. Choose complex carbs like whole grains, fruits, and veggies.

- Proteins: Help to build and repair tissues in the body. Choose lean proteins like chicken, fish, beans, and lentils.

- Fats: Provide essential fatty acids and help absorb vitamins A, D, E, and K. Avocado, almonds, seeds, and olive oil are examples of healthful fats.

2. Determine calorie needs:

Individuals undergoing treatment for leukaemia may have different calorie needs due to factors such as age, weight, activity level, and treatment side effects. Consult a registered dietitian or healthcare provider to determine the appropriate calorie intake for the individual.

3. Plan meals with a balance of macronutrients:

To balance macronutrients in every meal, aim for:

- **Carbohydrates:** 45-65% of total calories

- **Proteins:** 10-35% of total calories

- **Fats:** 20-35% of total calories

For example, a 1200-calorie meal plan might look like this:

Breakfast (450 calories):
- 1 cup oatmeal (170 calories) - complex carbohydrate
- 1 medium banana (105 calories) - complex carbohydrate and potassium source
- 1 hard-boiled egg (78 calories) - protein source
- 1 tablespoon almond butter (98 calories) - healthy fat source and added protein from nuts
- 1 cup unsweetened almond milk (30 calories) - low-calorie beverage option with added calcium and vitamin D from fortified almond milk
Total calories: 471 | Carbohydrates: 62g | Protein: 12g | Fat: 20g

Lunch (450 calories):
- 2 cups mixed greens (25 calories) - low calorie but high fibre source of carbohydrates and vitamins/minerals from greens like kale or spinach.
- ½ cup cooked quinoa (118 calories) - complex carbohydrate and added protein from quinoa seeds. - ½ cup grilled chicken breast (170 calories) - lean protein source with added iron from chicken breast. - ½ medium avocado (114 calories) - healthy fat source with added fibre from avocado skin. - 1 tablespoon olive oil dressing (67 calories) - healthy fat source with added flavour from olive oil dressing. Total calories: 424 | Carbohydrates: 38g | Protein: 26g | Fat: 23g

Dinner (450 calories):
- ½ cup cooked brown rice (218 calories) - complex carbohydrate with added fibre from brown rice bran.

- ½ cup baked salmon fillet (200 calories) - lean protein source with added omega-3 fatty acids from salmon fillet. - ½ cup steamed broccoli florets (34 calories) - low calorie but high fibre source of carbohydrates and vitamins/minerals from broccoli florets. - ½ medium orange (62 calories) - complex carbohydrate with added vitamin C from orange segments. Total calories: 416 | Carbohydrates: 49g | Protein: 27g | Fat: 16g

Snack options for between meals could include things like fresh fruit with a small handful of nuts or seeds or a small serving of Greek yoghourt with berries and a drizzle of honey or maple syrup for added sweetness without excess sugar or refined carbohydrates that can cause blood sugar spikes or crashes that can negatively impact energy levels during treatment for leukaemia patients. By following these guidelines for balancing macronutrients in every meal, individuals undergoing treatment for leukaemia can ensure they are meeting their nutritional needs while also managing symptoms such as fatigue and nausea that can make it challenging to eat enough throughout the day.

Creating Varied and Enjoyable Menus

Creating varied and enjoyable menus is essential in mindful meal planning for a leukaemia diet cookbook. Leukaemia patients undergoing chemotherapy or radiation therapy may experience side effects such as nausea, fatigue, and loss of appetite, making it challenging to consume enough nutrients to maintain a healthy body. A well-planned menu that is both nutritious and appealing can help alleviate these symptoms and promote a positive eating experience.

Here are some tips for creating varied and enjoyable menus in mindful meal planning for a leukaemia diet cookbook:

☐ Focus on Nutrient-Dense Foods: Leukaemia patients require foods that are rich in nutrients such as protein, iron, vitamins, and minerals. These foods will help them maintain a healthy weight, build muscle mass, and fight off infection. Some examples of nutrient-dense foods include lean meats, poultry, fish, legumes, whole grains, fruits, and vegetables.

☐ Incorporate Flavourful Spices and Herbs: Spices and herbs can add flavour to meals without adding excess salt or sugar. They also have medicinal properties that can help alleviate symptoms such as nausea and inflammation. Some examples of flavourful spices and herbs include ginger, turmeric, garlic, rosemary, thyme, and parsley.

☐ Use Healthy Fats: Healthy fats such as olive oil, avocado oil, nuts, seeds, and fatty fish can help the body absorb nutrients better and provide energy. They also contain omega-3 fatty acids that can help reduce inflammation.

- [ ] Include Fibre-Rich Foods: Fibre-rich foods such as whole grains, fruits, and vegetables can help prevent constipation, which is a common side effect of chemotherapy and radiation therapy. They also provide energy and promote a healthy digestive system.

- [ ] Offer Variety: Offering a variety of foods will prevent boredom and ensure that the patient is consuming a wide range of nutrients. This can include different types of proteins, grains, fruits, and vegetables.

- [ ] Consider Texture: Some leukaemia patients may experience mouth sores or difficulty swallowing due to treatment side effects. Offering soft or pureed foods can make it easier for them to eat without causing discomfort.

- [ ] Provide Small Meals: Eating small meals throughout the day instead of large meals can help alleviate nausea and prevent fatigue. This also allows the patient to consume more nutrients throughout the day instead of consuming large amounts at once.

- ☐ Encourage Hydration: Dehydration is a common side effect of chemotherapy and radiation therapy. Encouraging the patient to drink plenty of water throughout the day can help prevent dehydration and promote hydration before meals to aid in digestion.

By following these tips for creating varied and enjoyable menus in mindful meal planning for a leukaemia diet cookbook, you can provide nutritious meals that are both delicious and easy to consume for leukaemia patients undergoing treatment.

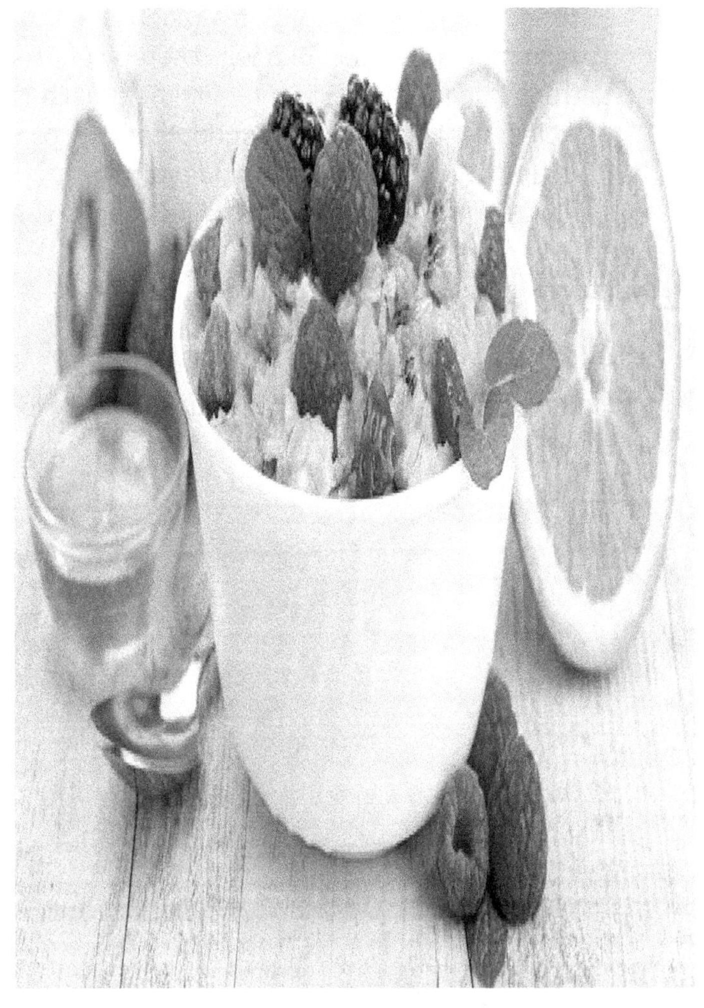

CHAPTER SEVEN

Resources and Additional Information

Helpful Tips for Grocery Shopping

Grocery shopping can be a daunting task, especially for individuals following a leukaemia diet. This diet is designed to support the body during cancer treatment and promote overall health. _Here are some helpful tips for grocery shopping to make the process easier and more efficient:_

1. Make a list:

Before you go shopping, make a list of the items you'll need. This will assist you in remaining focused and avoiding impulse purchases.

2. Plan your meals:

Take some time to plan your meals for the week ahead. This will help you determine which ingredients you need and prevent overbuying or underbuying.

3. Stick to the perimeter:

The outer edges of the grocery store typically contain fresh produce, meats, and dairy products. Try to shop primarily in these areas to avoid processed foods and added sugars.

4. Read labels:

Always read the labels of packaged foods to ensure they are leukaemia-friendly. Look for foods that are low in fat, sugar, and salt, and high in protein and fibre.

5. Choose whole grains:

Whole grains such as brown rice, quinoa, and whole wheat bread are rich in fibre and nutrients. They also help keep you fuller for longer periods of time.

6. Opt for lean proteins:

Lean proteins such as chicken, turkey, fish, and legumes are great sources of protein without adding excess fat or calories.

7. Limit processed foods:

Processed foods often contain added sugars, salt, and preservatives that can negatively impact your health. Try to limit your intake of processed foods and opt for whole, unprocessed foods instead.

8. Shop seasonally:

Fresh fruits and vegetables that are in season are typically less expensive and more flavorful than those that are out of season. They also tend to be more nutrient-dense since they don't have to travel as far to reach your grocery store.

9. Buy in bulk:

Purchasing items such as rice, beans, and nuts in bulk can save you money in the long run and reduce packaging waste. Just be sure to store them properly to prevent spoilage or contamination.

10. Don't forget about hydration:

Drinking plenty of water is essential for maintaining good health during cancer treatment. Be sure to bring a reusable water bottle with you to the grocery store to stay hydrated throughout your shopping trip.

By following these tips, you can make grocery shopping a more efficient and enjoyable experience while also supporting your health during cancer treatment. Remember to always consult with your healthcare provider for specific dietary recommendations based on your individual needs and treatment plan.

Links to Further Reading and Supportive Organizations

At the end of our Leukaemia diet Cookbook, we have included a section dedicated to providing links to further reading and supportive organisations. This section is designed to provide our readers with additional resources and information related to leukaemia and its treatment, as well as support for those affected by this disease.

Further Reading:

1. Leukaemia Foundation
- The Leukaemia Foundation is a leading organisation in Australia that provides information, resources, and support for people affected by leukaemia, lymphoma, and myeloma. Their website offers a wealth of information on leukaemia, including treatment options, lifestyle tips, and research updates.

2. Cancer Council Australia
- The Cancer Council Australia is a national organisation that provides information, support, and advocacy for people affected by cancer. Their website offers a range of resources related to

leukaemia, including information on treatment options, clinical trials, and lifestyle tips.

3. American Cancer Society

- The American Cancer Society is a leading organisation in the United States that provides information, resources, and support for people affected by cancer. Their website offers a range of resources related to leukaemia, including information on treatment options, clinical trials, and lifestyle tips.

Supportive Organisations:

1. Leukaemia Foundation

- As mentioned earlier, the Leukaemia Foundation is a leading organisation in Australia that provides information, resources, and support for people affected by leukaemia, lymphoma, and myeloma. They offer a range of support services, including patient support programs, financial assistance programs, and accommodation services for people travelling to treatment centres.

2. Cancer Council Australia

- The Cancer Council Australia provides a range of support services for people affected by cancer, including information and support services for patients and their families, as well as advocacy and research initiatives aimed at improving cancer outcomes

<u>*3. American Cancer Society*</u>
- The American Cancer Society offers a range of support services for people affected by cancer, including patient support programs, financial assistance programs, and accommodation services for people travelling to treatment centres. They also offer a range of resources related to nutrition and healthy eating during cancer treatment.

We hope that these resources will be helpful to our readers in their journey towards managing leukaemia through dietary changes. Remember to always consult with your healthcare team before making any significant changes to your diet or treatment plan.

CONCLUSION

Maintaining a Healthy Diet During Leukaemia Treatment

The Importance of Continuing Good Nutrition Habits

Leukaemia is a type of cancer that affects the blood-forming cells in the bone marrow. The treatment for leukaemia can be intense and often includes chemotherapy, radiation therapy, and bone marrow transplantation. While these treatments are essential for managing the disease, they can also take a toll on a person's overall health and wellbeing, particularly their nutrition.

Maintaining good nutrition habits during leukaemia treatment is crucial for managing symptoms, reducing side effects, and promoting overall health. Here are some reasons why continuing good nutrition habits is important during leukaemia treatment:

Managing Symptoms:

Leukaemia treatment can cause a range of symptoms, including nausea, vomiting, loss of appetite, and mouth sores. Eating small, frequent meals throughout the day can help manage these symptoms by keeping the stomach full and preventing nausea. Choosing foods that are easy to digest, such as cooked vegetables, fruits, and whole-grain breads, can also help prevent further discomfort.

Chemotherapy and radiation therapy can cause a range of side effects, including fatigue, diarrhoea, and weight loss. Eating a balanced diet with plenty of protein can help prevent muscle loss and maintain energy levels. Choosing foods rich in fibre can also help prevent diarrhoea by promoting regular bowel movements.

Leukaemia treatment can weaken the immune system, making it more susceptible to infection. Eating a diet rich in vitamins and minerals can help support overall health and promote a strong immune system. Foods rich in vitamin C, such as citrus fruits and bell peppers, can help promote wound healing and reduce inflammation. Foods rich in iron, such as red meat and leafy greens, can help prevent anaemia, which is common during leukaemia treatment due to decreased red blood cell production.

Eating healthy foods during leukaemia treatment can also help promote a positive attitude and outlook on life. Choosing foods that are enjoyable and satisfying can help reduce stress and promote feelings of wellbeing. Engaging in cooking activities with loved ones or participating in cooking classes can also provide a sense of normalcy and control during an otherwise uncertain time.

In conclusion, maintaining good nutrition habits during leukaemia treatment is essential for managing symptoms, reducing side effects, promoting overall health, and maintaining a positive attitude. Working with a registered dietitian or healthcare provider to develop a personalised nutrition plan can provide additional guidance on how to make healthy choices during this challenging time. By prioritising nutrition throughout leukaemia treatment, individuals can improve their overall health and wellbeing while managing the disease.

Resources for Further Information

Leukaemia is a blood malignancy that affects the bone marrow. Treatment for leukaemia can be intense and often involves chemotherapy, radiation therapy, and stem cell transplants. These treatments can take a toll on the body, making it important for individuals with leukaemia to maintain a healthy diet to support their overall health and wellbeing during treatment.

Here are some resources for further information on maintaining a healthy diet during leukaemia treatment:

1. Leukaemia Foundation of Australia
- Nutrition and Leukaemia: This resource provides information on the importance of nutrition during leukaemia treatment, as well as tips for managing common side effects. Treatment side effects include nausea, vomiting, and mouth sores. It also includes a list of foods to eat and avoid during treatment.

2. American Cancer Society
- Nutrition During Cancer Treatment: This resource provides general information on the importance of nutrition during cancer treatment, including tips for managing side effects such as fatigue, loss of appetite, and weight loss. It also includes information on specific nutrients that may be beneficial during treatment, such as protein and vitamin D.

3. National Cancer Institute
- Nutrition During Cancer Treatment: This resource provides detailed information on the role of nutrition during cancer treatment, including tips for managing common side effects such as taste changes, mouth sores, and diarrhoea. It also includes information on specific nutrients that may

be beneficial during treatment, such as omega-3 fatty acids and antioxidants.

4. Cancer Research UK
- Eating Well During Cancer Treatment: This resource provides practical tips for maintaining a healthy diet during cancer treatment, including suggestions for meal planning and food preparation. It also includes information on how to manage common side effects such as fatigue and taste changes.

5. Leukaemia & Lymphoma Society
- Nutrition During Treatment: This resource provides detailed information on the role of nutrition during leukaemia treatment, including tips for managing common side effects such as nausea, vomiting, and mouth sores. It also includes information on specific nutrients that may be beneficial during treatment, such as protein and vitamin B12.

These resources provide valuable information for individuals with leukaemia who are undergoing treatment. By following the tips and advice provided in these resources, individuals can help support their overall health and wellbeing during this challenging time.

Encouragement to Stay Positive and Focus on Wellness

Leukaemia is a cancer that affects the blood and bone marrow, making it challenging for patients to maintain a healthy diet during treatment. Chemotherapy and radiation therapy, which are common treatments for leukaemia, can cause side effects such as nausea, vomiting, and loss of appetite, making it difficult for patients to consume enough nutrients to support their bodies. However, it's essential to encourage leukaemia patients to stay positive and focus on wellness by maintaining a healthy diet during treatment.

Firstly, a healthy diet can help patients manage the side effects of treatment. For instance, foods rich in protein such as lean meats, eggs, and beans can help prevent muscle loss caused by chemotherapy. Foods high in fibre such as whole grains, fruits, and vegetables can also help prevent constipation caused by opioid pain medication commonly used during treatment.

Secondly, a healthy diet can boost the immune system, which is crucial for leukaemia patients undergoing treatment. Leukaemia affects the production of white blood cells, which are essential for fighting infections. A diet rich in vitamin C-containing foods such as citrus fruits and bell peppers can help boost the immune system. Additionally, foods rich in zinc such as oysters, pumpkin seeds, and beans can also help boost the immune system.

Thirdly, a healthy diet can improve overall well-being during treatment. Eating small frequent meals instead of large meals can help prevent nausea and vomiting caused by chemotherapy. Additionally, drinking plenty of water can help prevent dehydration caused by diarrhoea or vomiting.

Encouraging leukaemia patients to stay positive and focus on wellness during treatment is essential. Patients may feel overwhelmed and discouraged by the side effects of treatment; however, reminding them of the benefits of a healthy diet can help them stay motivated. Here are some tips for encouraging patients to maintain a healthy diet during leukaemia treatment:

1. Consult with a registered dietitian:

A registered dietitian can provide personalised nutrition advice based on the patient's specific needs during treatment. They can also provide tips on how to manage side effects such as nausea and loss of appetite.

2. Encourage small frequent meals:

Eating small frequent meals instead of large meals can help prevent nausea and vomiting caused by chemotherapy. Patients should aim to eat six small meals a day instead of three large meals.

3. Focus on nutrient-dense foods:

Patients should aim to consume foods that are high in nutrients such as protein, fibre, vitamins, and minerals to support their bodies during treatment. Foods such as lean meats, eggs, whole grains, fruits, and vegetables are excellent sources of these nutrients.

4. Stay hydrated:

Dehydration is common during leukaemia treatment due to diarrhoea or vomiting; therefore, it's essential to drink plenty of water throughout the day to prevent dehydration. Patients should aim to drink at least eight glasses of water a day.

5. Limit processed foods:

Processed foods such as fast food and packaged snacks are often high in salt, sugar, and unhealthy fats that can negatively impact overall health during treatment. Patients should aim to limit their intake of processed foods and focus on whole foods instead.

In conclusion, encouraging leukaemia patients to stay positive and focus on wellness during treatment is essential. Maintaining a healthy diet can help manage side effects such as nausea and loss of appetite while also boosting the immune system and improving overall well-being during treatment. By consulting with a registered dietitian, focusing on nutrient-dense foods, staying hydrated, limiting processed foods, and eating small frequent meals, patients can maintain a healthy diet during leukaemia treatment while also supporting their bodies through this challenging time.

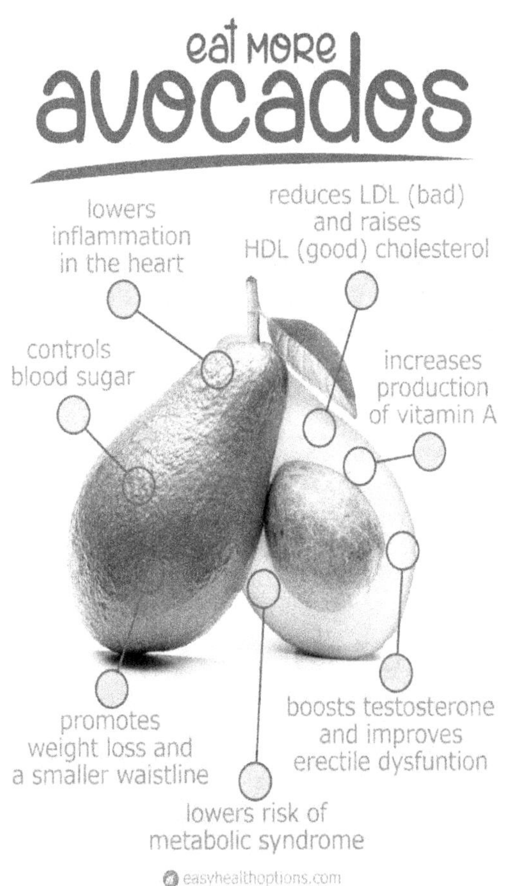

eat MORe
avocados
lowers inflammation in the heart
reduces LDL (bad) and raises HDL (good) cholesterol
controls blood sugar
increases production of vitamin A
promotes weight loss and a smaller waistline
boosts testosterone and improves erectile dysfuntion
lowers risk of metabolic syndrome
easyhealthoptions.com

www.ingramcontent.com/pod-product-compliance
Lightning Source LLC
Chambersburg PA
CBHW061004260726
48661CB00005B/2055